Unlocking Your Inner Vitality

The Transformative Power of the Lipocaloric Diet

BY
Lucy Scott

Disclaimer

Copyright © by Lucy Scott 2023.
All rights reserved.

Table of contents

Introduction

In today's fast-paced world, where convenience and processed foods often take precedence over mindful eating, achieving optimal health and well-being can seem like an elusive goal. We are bombarded with conflicting dietary advice, and the path to a healthier lifestyle can feel overwhelming and confusing.

The Lipocaloric Diet offers a transformative approach to nutrition and well-being, empowering you to take control of your health and unlock your true potential. This comprehensive guide will equip you with the knowledge and tools you need to embark on a journey of profound transformation, one that extends beyond weight loss and encompasses holistic well-being.

At the heart of the Lipocaloric Diet lies the concept of nutrient density, a powerful approach to eating that prioritizes nutrient-rich foods while minimizing calorie intake. By focusing on whole, unprocessed foods, you provide your body with the essential nutrients it needs to function optimally, while simultaneously reducing the consumption of empty calories that can lead to weight gain and chronic health issues.

The Lipocaloric Diet is not merely a restrictive diet; it is a holistic approach to well-being that encompasses physical, mental, and emotional health. You will learn how to incorporate regular physical activity, effective stress management techniques, and mindful living practices into your daily routine, creating a synergistic effect that promotes overall well-being and enhances your quality of life.

This book will guide you through every step of the Lipocaloric journey, from understanding the science behind the diet to implementing practical strategies for achieving your health goals. You will discover:

The principles of nutrient-dense eating and how to make informed food choices

Effective strategies for incorporating physical activity into your lifestyle

Practical techniques for managing stress and fostering emotional well-being

Mindful living practices to enhance your overall well-being

Recipes and meal plans tailored to the Lipocaloric Diet

Guidance on navigating challenges and maintaining success

The Lipocaloric Diet is not a quick fix or a temporary solution; it is a lifelong commitment to nourishing your body and mind. As you embark on this transformative journey, you will discover a profound sense of empowerment, embracing a healthier lifestyle that aligns with your values and aspirations.

Embrace the Lipocaloric Diet, and unlock a world of vitality, well-being, and limitless possibilities

Part 1

Introduction to the Lipocaloric Diet

Chapter 1

The Lipocaloric Revolution: Unveiling the Secrets of a Health-Transforming Diet

In the realm of nutrition, a revolution is brewing, one that has the potential to transform lives and redefine our understanding of wellness. The Lipocaloric Diet, a groundbreaking approach to achieving optimal health and preventing chronic disease, stands at the forefront of this transformation. This chapter delves into the essence of the Lipocaloric

Diet, unveiling the secrets behind its remarkable effectiveness and transformative power.

The Essence of Lipocalorics: A Paradigm Shift in Nutrition

The Lipocaloric Diet is a revolutionary dietary strategy that challenges conventional dietary wisdom. It is characterized by its focus on calorie restriction and nutrient density, emphasizing the consumption of whole, unprocessed foods while minimizing calorie intake. This unique approach stands in stark contrast to the abundance of high-calorie, low-nutrient foods that dominate modern diets.

The Science Behind Lipocalorics: Unveiling the Mechanisms of Metabolic Transformation

The Lipocaloric Diet's remarkable effectiveness stems from its profound impact on cellular metabolism. By reducing calorie intake while maintaining high nutrient intake, the body is forced to adapt its energy production pathways. This metabolic shift, known as metabolic adaptation, leads to a cascade of positive effects, including:

- **Enhanced fat burning:** The body begins to utilize stored fat for energy more efficiently, leading to significant weight loss.

- **Improved insulin sensitivity**: Lipocalorics promote insulin sensitivity, enhancing the body's ability to regulate blood sugar levels and prevent the development of type 2 diabetes.

- **Reduced inflammation:** Inflammation, a root cause of many chronic diseases, is significantly reduced on the Lipocaloric Diet.

- Cellular rejuvenation: Lipocalorics trigger cellular autophagy, a process that cleans up damaged cells and promotes cellular renewal.

The Benefits of Lipocalorics: A Journey Beyond Weight Loss

The Lipocaloric Diet offers a multitude of benefits that extend far beyond weight loss. These benefits include:

- **Reduced risk of chronic diseases:** Lipocalorics have been shown to effectively prevent and even reverse chronic diseases such as type 2 diabetes, heart disease, and certain types of cancer.

- **Improved cognitive function:** Studies have demonstrated that the Lipocaloric Diet can enhance cognitive function, memory, and overall brain health.

- **Increased energy levels:** By optimizing cellular metabolism, Lipocalorics provide a sustained boost in energy levels throughout the day.

- **Enhanced well-being:** Lipocalorics have been associated with improved mood, reduced stress levels, and a greater sense of overall well-being.

Addressing Common Misconceptions: Dispelling Myths and Setting the Record Straight

The Lipocaloric Diet, with its emphasis on calorie restriction and a focus on nutrient-dense whole foods, has challenged conventional dietary wisdom and sparked various misconceptions. This chapter addresses common myths and sets the record straight about Lipocaloric nutrition, dispelling doubts and providing a clear understanding of this revolutionary dietary approach.

Myth 1: Lipocalorics Are Crash Diets

A common misconception is that Lipocalorics are akin to crash diets, characterized by extreme calorie restriction and a focus on quick weight loss. This is far from accurate. Lipocalorics emphasize a moderate reduction in calorie intake, ensuring that the body receives adequate nutrition while promoting sustainable weight loss and improved metabolic health. Crash diets, on the other hand, often lead to nutrient deficiencies, muscle loss, and a rebound effect upon returning to normal eating habits.

Myth 2: Lipocalorics Cause Muscle Loss

Another misconception is that Lipocalorics lead to significant muscle loss, particularly during weight loss phases. While some muscle loss may occur during initial weight loss, Lipocalorics can be tailored to minimize muscle loss and even promote muscle growth through proper protein intake and resistance training. In contrast, crash diets often result in significant muscle loss due to extreme calorie restriction and inadequate protein intake.

Myth 3: Lipocalorics Are Restrictive and Unsustainable

The notion that Lipocalorics are overly restrictive and unsustainable is often perpetuated. In reality, Lipocalorics promote a balanced and flexible approach to nutrition, emphasizing a variety of whole, unprocessed foods. This dietary approach can be easily adapted to individual preferences and lifestyles, making it sustainable for long-term success. Crash diets, on the other hand, are often characterized by strict rules and limitations, making them difficult to adhere to and leading to unsustainable weight loss practices.

Myth 4: Lipocalorics Are Only for Weight Loss

While weight loss is a primary focus of the Lipocaloric Diet, its benefits extend far beyond weight management. Lipocalorics have been shown to effectively prevent and even reverse chronic diseases such as type 2 diabetes, heart disease, and certain types of cancer. Additionally, Lipocalorics have been associated with improved cognitive function, increased energy levels, and enhanced overall well-being. Crash diets, on the other hand, primarily focus on quick weight loss and often lack the comprehensive benefits associated with Lipocalorics.

Myth 5: Lipocalorics Require Professional Supervision

While professional guidance can be beneficial, Lipocalorics can be successfully implemented without constant supervision. With access to reliable information and a commitment to healthy eating, individuals can adopt Lipocalorics principles and achieve remarkable health outcomes. Crash diets, on the other hand, often require strict adherence to a predetermined plan and may require professional supervision to prevent potential health risks.

Setting the Record Straight: Embracing Lipocalorics for a Healthier Future

Setting the record straight about Lipocalorics is crucial to dispel misconceptions and promote a deeper understanding of this revolutionary dietary approach. Lipocalorics, when implemented correctly, offer a safe, effective, and sustainable path to achieving optimal health and preventing chronic disease. By embracing Lipocalorics and dispelling the myths that surround it, individuals can embark on a journey towards a healthier, happier, and more fulfilling life.

Chapter 2

Understanding the Science Behind Lipocalorics: A Deep Dive into the Metabolic Mechanisms

The Lipocaloric Diet, with its profound impact on cellular metabolism, stands as a testament to the intricate workings of the human body. To fully grasp the transformative power of this dietary approach, we must embark on a deep dive into the metabolic mechanisms that underpin its success. This chapter will unravel the scientific underpinnings of Lipocalorics, revealing the remarkable processes that drive weight loss, metabolic optimization, and overall health improvement.

Calorie Restriction: Triggering Metabolic Adaptation

The cornerstone of the Lipocaloric Diet is a moderate reduction in daily calorie intake. This controlled calorie restriction, far from being a mere reduction in food intake, triggers a series of metabolic adaptations that promote weight loss and overall health.

Metabolic Switching: From Glucose to Fat Burning

When calorie intake is reduced, the body shifts from relying primarily on glucose, derived from carbohydrates, for energy to utilizing stored fat reserves. This metabolic switch, known as ketosis, is a hallmark of the Lipocaloric Diet and plays a crucial role in its effectiveness.

During ketosis, the liver breaks down stored fat into fatty acids, which are then converted into ketones, an alternative energy source for the body. This metabolic shift leads to several beneficial effects:

- **Efficient fat burning:** Ketones provide a more efficient source of energy than glucose, leading to enhanced fat burning and weight loss.

- **Reduced appetite:** Ketones suppress the appetite-stimulating hormone ghrelin, contributing to reduced calorie intake and sustained weight loss.

- **Preserved muscle mass:** Ketones provide an alternative energy source for muscles, preventing muscle loss during weight loss phases.

Hormonal Symphony: Orchestrating Metabolic Harmony

Lipocalorics not only influence metabolic pathways but also exert a profound impact on the body's hormonal milieu. By regulating key hormones involved in appetite control, metabolism, and energy expenditure, Lipocalorics create an environment conducive to weight loss and metabolic optimization.

- **Insulin sensitivity:** Lipocalorics promote insulin sensitivity, enabling the body to effectively utilize glucose for energy and prevent blood sugar spikes. This improved insulin sensitivity is crucial for preventing type 2 diabetes and other metabolic disorders.

- **Leptin signaling:** Leptin, the satiety hormone, signals the brain when the body has stored enough energy. Lipocalorics enhance leptin signaling, leading to a reduced appetite and increased satiety, thereby facilitating weight management.

- **Cortisol regulation:** Cortisol, a stress hormone, can promote fat storage. Lipocalorics help regulate cortisol levels, reducing its negative impact on metabolism.

Cellular Rejuvenation: Autophagy's Role in Renewal

Calorie restriction, a core principle of the Lipocaloric Diet, activates cellular autophagy, a process that removes damaged cellular components and promotes cell renewal. This cellular rejuvenation process plays a critical role in maintaining optimal cellular function and preventing age-related diseases.

Autophagy, often referred to as the body's cellular recycling system, targets damaged proteins, organelles, and cellular debris, clearing the way for the production of new, functional cellular components. This process not only enhances cellular health but also contributes to weight loss and metabolic optimization.

The Role of Nutrient Density: Fueling Cellular Vitality

While calorie restriction plays a crucial role in the Lipocaloric Diet, nutrient density is equally important. By emphasizing whole, unprocessed foods, the Lipocaloric Diet ensures that the body receives an abundance of essential vitamins, minerals, and antioxidants. These nutrients are vital for optimal cellular function, disease prevention, and overall well-being.

Micronutrient Powerhouse: Whole foods are packed with micronutrients, including vitamins, minerals, and phytochemicals, that play a myriad of roles in maintaining health and preventing chronic diseases. For instance, vitamin D enhances calcium absorption for bone health, while antioxidants combat oxidative stress, a major contributor to aging and chronic disease development.

Synergy of Calorie Restriction and Nutrient Density: A Double-Edged Sword for Health

The remarkable effectiveness of the Lipocaloric Diet stems from the synergistic interplay between calorie restriction and nutrient density. By simultaneously reducing calorie intake and maximizing nutrient intake, this dietary approach achieves a profound impact on cellular metabolism, leading to a cascade of health benefits.

- **Weight loss and metabolic optimization:** The combined effects of calorie restriction and nutrient density promote efficient fat burning, improved insulin sensitivity, and reduced inflammation, all of which contribute to successful weight loss and metabolic optimization.

- **Disease prevention and longevity:** Nutrient density provides the body with the essential tools to combat chronic diseases, while calorie restriction slows down the aging process, promoting longevity.

The Lipocaloric Diet and Chronic Disease Prevention

The Lipocaloric Diet's remarkable impact extends far beyond weight loss, offering significant protection against a wide range of chronic diseases. This chapter explores the specific mechanisms by which Lipocalorics prevent and even reverse chronic ailments, highlighting the far-reaching benefits of this revolutionary dietary approach.

Type 2 Diabetes: Reversing Insulin Resistance

Type 2 diabetes, characterized by elevated blood sugar levels due to insulin resistance, is a major public health concern. The Lipocaloric Diet has been shown to effectively reverse type 2 diabetes by improving insulin sensitivity and reducing blood sugar levels.

The underlying mechanism behind this remarkable effect lies in the combined impact of calorie restriction and nutrient density on insulin signaling. Calorie restriction promotes the production of adiponectin, a hormone that enhances insulin sensitivity.

Additionally, the abundance of micronutrients in Lipocalorics further supports insulin signaling and glucose uptake by cells.

Heart Disease: Protecting the Cardiovascular System

Heart disease, the leading cause of death worldwide, is directly linked to metabolic dysfunction and chronic inflammation. The Lipocaloric Diet has been demonstrated to protect against heart disease by improving cholesterol levels, reducing blood pressure, and decreasing inflammation.

The beneficial effects of Lipocalorics on heart health can be attributed to several factors, including:

- **Reduced LDL (bad) cholesterol and increased HDL (good) cholesterol:** Lipocalorics promote a shift in cholesterol levels, reducing the risk of atherosclerosis, a hardening of the arteries.

- **Lower blood pressure:** Calorie restriction and nutrient density contribute to lowering blood pressure, reducing the strain on the cardiovascular system.

- **Decreased inflammation:** Lipocalorics' anti-inflammatory properties help combat chronic inflammation, a major contributor to cardiovascular disease.

Neurological Disorders: Enhancing Brain Health

Neurological disorders, such as Alzheimer's disease and Parkinson's disease, pose a significant challenge to aging populations. The Lipocaloric Diet has demonstrated neuroprotective effects, potentially preventing or delaying the onset of these debilitating conditions.

Benefits of Lipocalorics on Brain Health

The benefits of Lipocalorics on brain health can be attributed to several mechanisms, including:

Increased ketone production: Ketones, produced during ketosis, provide an alternative energy source for the brain and may protect against neurodegeneration.

Reduced oxidative stress: Lipocalorics' antioxidant properties help combat oxidative stress, a major factor in neurological damage.

Enhanced brain-derived neurotrophic factor (BDNF) production: BDNF, a neuroprotective protein, is crucial for maintaining brain health and may be stimulated by Lipocalorics.

Cancer Prevention: Combating Cellular Malignancy

Cancer, a leading cause of death worldwide, is characterized by uncontrolled cellular growth. The Lipocaloric Diet has been linked to reduced cancer risk, potentially stemming from its impact on cellular metabolism and inflammation.

The cancer-preventive effects of Lipocalorics may be attributed to several factors, including:

Reduced insulin levels: Chronic high insulin levels are associated with increased cancer risk. Lipocalorics help regulate insulin levels, potentially lowering cancer risk.

Suppressed inflammation: Chronic inflammation promotes cancer development. Lipocalorics' anti-inflammatory properties may help combat cancer.

Enhanced DNA repair: DNA damage is a precursor to cancer. Lipocalorics may promote DNA repair mechanisms, reducing cancer risk.

Conclusion: Unveiling a Path to Optimal Health

The Lipocaloric Diet, with its profound impact on cellular metabolism, stands as a powerful tool for achieving optimal health and preventing chronic disease. By understanding the intricate mechanisms behind this revolutionary dietary approach, we can harness its transformative power to enhance our well-being and lead healthier, longer lives.

Chapter 3

Embracing the Lipocaloric Lifestyle: Implementing the Diet for Optimal Health and Wellness

The Lipocaloric Diet, with its profound impact on cellular metabolism and its far-reaching health benefits, offers a transformative path to optimal health and wellness. Embracing the Lipocaloric lifestyle requires a holistic approach that encompasses not only dietary choices but also lifestyle habits and mindset shifts.

This chapter delves into the practical aspects of implementing the Lipocaloric Diet, providing a comprehensive guide to navigating this transformative approach to nutrition.

Understanding Your Body's Unique Needs: Tailoring the Lipocaloric Diet

The Lipocaloric Diet is not a one-size-fits-all approach. Each individual possesses unique metabolic needs and lifestyle factors that influence their response to the diet. Tailoring the Lipocaloric Diet to individual needs is crucial for achieving optimal results and ensuring long-term success.

Identifying Your Calorie Needs:

The starting point for implementing the Lipocaloric Diet is determining your daily calorie needs. This involves calculating your basal metabolic rate (BMR), which represents the energy your body expends at rest, and factoring in your activity level. Once your calorie needs are established, a moderate reduction, typically around 20-30%, is recommended to initiate weight loss.

Prioritizing Nutrient Density:

While calorie restriction plays a vital role in the Lipocaloric Diet, nutrient density is equally important. Emphasizing whole, unprocessed foods, such as fruits, vegetables, legumes, whole grains, and lean protein sources, ensures that the body receives an abundance of essential vitamins, minerals, and antioxidants. These nutrients are vital for optimal cellular function, disease prevention, and overall well-being.

Personalizing Meal Planning:

The Lipocaloric Diet is not about strict meal plans or rigid restrictions. Instead, it encourages a flexible approach that allows for individual preferences and dietary needs. Meal planning can be simplified by incorporating a variety of nutrient-dense foods and portion control strategies.

Mindful Eating Practices:

Mindful eating is an essential component of the Lipocaloric lifestyle. It involves paying attention to hunger cues, eating slowly, savoring flavors, and avoiding distractions while eating. Mindful eating promotes satiety, prevents overeating, and enhances the overall dining experience.

Embracing Lifestyle Habits for Enhanced Well-being:

The Lipocaloric Diet goes beyond dietary choices, encompassing a holistic approach to well-being. Integrating healthy lifestyle habits into the Lipocaloric journey amplifies its benefits and promotes overall well-being.

Regular Physical Activity:

Regular physical activity is an integral part of the Lipocaloric lifestyle. Exercise not only enhances weight loss but also improves cardiovascular health, boosts energy levels, and promotes muscle maintenance. Aim for at least 30 minutes of moderate-intensity exercise most days of the week.

Adequate Sleep:

Sleep plays a crucial role in regulating metabolism, hormones, and overall health. Aim for 7-8 hours of quality sleep each night to optimize your body's functioning and maximize the benefits of the Lipocaloric Diet.

Stress Management:

Chronic stress can negatively impact metabolism and hinder weight loss efforts. Incorporate stress-management techniques such as yoga, meditation, or spending time in nature into your routine to promote relaxation and overall well-being.

Mindset Shifts for Sustainable Success:

Adopting a positive mindset and cultivating a growth-oriented approach are essential for long-term success with the Lipocaloric Diet.

Embracing a Journey, Not a Destination:

The Lipocaloric Diet is a journey, not a race. View it as a process of gradual change and embrace the learning experience along the way. Celebrate small victories, learn from setbacks, and maintain a positive outlook.

Seeking Support and Guidance:

Don't hesitate to seek support from healthcare professionals, registered dietitians, or online communities to gain personalized guidance and encouragement throughout your Lipocaloric journey.

Conclusion: Embracing a Healthier, Happier You

The Lipocaloric Diet, when embraced with a holistic approach and a positive mindset, offers a transformative path to achieving optimal health and wellness. By understanding your unique needs, tailoring your diet, incorporating healthy lifestyle habits, and cultivating a growth-oriented mindset, you can unlock the remarkable benefits of Lipocalorics and embark on a journey towards a healthier, happier you

Part 2

The Lipocaloric Diet: A Comprehensive Guide

Chapter 4

Tailoring Your Lipocaloric Experience: Personalizing the Diet to Fit Your Unique Needs

The Lipocaloric Diet, with its emphasis on calorie restriction and nutrient density, offers a revolutionary approach to achieving optimal health and preventing chronic disease. However, the effectiveness of this dietary strategy hinges on its ability to be tailored to individual needs and preferences. This chapter delves into the art of personalizing the Lipocaloric Diet, ensuring that it seamlessly integrates into your unique lifestyle and maximizes its transformative impact.

Unearthing Your Unique Metabolic Fingerprint

Every individual possesses a unique metabolic fingerprint, a combination of genetic predispositions, lifestyle factors, and environmental influences that shapes their response to the Lipocaloric Diet. Unraveling this metabolic fingerprint is crucial for customizing the diet to maximize its effectiveness.

Assessing Your Basal Metabolic Rate (BMR):

The BMR represents the energy your body expends at rest, providing a baseline for determining your daily calorie needs. Calculating your BMR involves considering factors such as age, gender, height, and weight.

Gauging Your Activity Level:

Physical activity plays a significant role in overall calorie expenditure. Accurately assessing your activity level, whether through fitness trackers or self-monitoring, is essential for tailoring your calorie intake.

Identifying Dietary Sensitivities and Allergies:

Certain foods may trigger sensitivities or allergies, causing digestive issues and hindering weight loss efforts. Identifying and avoiding these foods is crucial for a personalized Lipocaloric approach.

Considering Cultural and Culinary Preferences:

The Lipocaloric Diet should not be a departure from your cultural and culinary preferences. Instead, it should be adapted to incorporate the flavors, traditions, and ingredients that align with your heritage and taste buds.

Tailoring Macronutrient Ratios:

The Lipocaloric Diet is not a one-size-fits-all macronutrient plan. The optimal ratio of carbohydrates, proteins, and fats depends on individual factors such as activity level, muscle mass, and personal preferences.

Accommodating Dietary Restrictions and Preferences:

The Lipocaloric Diet can be successfully implemented with various dietary restrictions, such as vegetarian, vegan, or gluten-free. It is crucial to find nutrient-dense alternatives within these restrictions to ensure adequate nutrition.

Harnessing Technology for Personalized Guidance:

Numerous online tools and mobile applications can assist in tailoring the Lipocaloric Diet to individual needs. These tools can provide personalized meal plans, track calorie intake, and offer support and guidance throughout the journey.

Embracing Flexibility and Adaptability

The Lipocaloric Diet should not be a rigid or inflexible regimen. It should be adaptable to accommodate social events, travel, or unexpected changes in routine. Flexibility promotes long-term adherence and reduces the risk of burnout.

Consulting with Healthcare Professionals:

Seeking guidance from healthcare professionals, such as registered dietitians or physicians, can provide valuable insights into personalizing the Lipocaloric Diet. They can assess individual needs, address specific concerns, and recommend appropriate adaptations.

Conclusion: Unveiling Your Personalized Lipocaloric Path

Personalizing the Lipocaloric Diet is an ongoing journey of exploration and self-discovery. By understanding your unique metabolic fingerprint, tailoring macronutrient ratios, accommodating dietary preferences, and embracing flexibility, you can transform the Lipocaloric Diet into a powerful tool for achieving optimal health and wellness. Remember, the key lies in finding a balance between scientific principles and personal preferences, creating a dietary approach that seamlessly integrates into your life and nurtures your well-being.

Chapter 5

Unleashing the Power of Nutrient Density: Fueling Your Body with Whole, Unprocessed Foods

The Lipocaloric Diet, with its emphasis on calorie restriction, goes beyond mere calorie counting and delves into the realm of nutrient density. By prioritizing nutrient-rich whole foods, this dietary approach ensures that the body receives an abundance of essential vitamins, minerals, and antioxidants, laying the foundation for optimal health and disease prevention. This chapter explores the concept of nutrient density and its profound impact on the Lipocaloric journey.

Embracing Whole Foods: The Cornerstone of Nutrient Density

Whole foods, unprocessed and minimally altered from their natural state, are the cornerstone of nutrient density. They are packed with essential vitamins, minerals, phytochemicals, and fiber, all of which play crucial roles in maintaining cellular function, preventing chronic diseases, and promoting overall well-being.

Fruits and Vegetables: Nature's Multivitamin

Fruits and vegetables are nature's multivitamins, offering a kaleidoscope of nutrients that support various bodily functions. They are rich in antioxidants, which combat oxidative stress and reduce the risk of chronic diseases. Fruits and vegetables also provide fiber, essential for digestive health and satiety.

Legumes and Whole Grains: Protein Powerhouses

Legumes, such as beans, lentils, and peas, are excellent sources of plant-based protein, fiber, and essential minerals. Whole grains, including brown rice, quinoa, and oats, provide complex carbohydrates, fiber, and a range of vitamins and minerals.

Lean Protein Sources: Building Blocks for Body and Mind

Lean protein sources, such as chicken, fish, eggs, and tofu, are crucial for maintaining muscle mass, supporting tissue repair, and providing the building blocks for neurotransmitters and hormones.

Healthy Fats: Essential for Cellular Function

Healthy fats, found in sources such as avocados, nuts, seeds, and olive oil, play a vital role in cellular function, hormone production, and nutrient absorption. They also contribute to satiety and promote brain health.

Limiting Processed Foods: A Path to Nutrient Deprivation

Processed foods, often high in calories, unhealthy fats, added sugars, and sodium, contribute to nutrient deprivation and increase the risk of chronic diseases. They offer little nutritional value and can hinder weight loss efforts.

Decoding Food Labels: Navigating the Nutritional Landscape

Understanding food labels is essential for making informed choices and ensuring that your Lipocaloric journey is fueled by nutrient-dense foods. Pay attention to serving sizes, nutrient percentages, and ingredient lists to prioritize whole, unprocessed options.

Meal Planning and Preparation: Simplifying Nutrient-Rich Eating

Planning your meals in advance and preparing nutrient-dense snacks can simplify healthy eating and prevent last-minute unhealthy choices. This approach also helps you track your calorie intake and ensure you're getting a variety of nutrients throughout the day.

Cooking with Care: Preserving Nutritional Value

Cooking methods can significantly impact nutrient retention. Opt for steaming, baking, grilling, or poaching to preserve the nutritional integrity of your food choices. Avoid deep-frying and excessive use of added fats and sugars.

Conclusion: Nourishing Your Body with Nutrient-Dense Abundance

By embracing whole, unprocessed foods and limiting processed options, you transform the Lipocaloric Diet into a nutrient-dense journey that nourishes your body and optimizes your health. Remember, nutrient density is not about restriction but about providing your body with the essential building blocks for optimal function and long-term well-being

Chapter 6

Embracing a Mindful Approach to Eating: Enhancing Satiety and Enjoyment

Mindful eating, a cornerstone of the Lipocaloric Diet, goes beyond mere calorie counting and delves into the realm of conscious awareness and appreciation for food. It is a practice that promotes satiety, deepens the connection between mind and body, and transforms mealtimes into moments of mindfulness and enjoyment.

The Essence of Mindful Eating: Cultivating a Conscious Connection with Food

Mindful eating is not about deprivation or restriction; it is about cultivating a conscious connection with food and eating. It involves paying attention to internal hunger cues, savoring flavors, and appreciating the sensory experience of nourishment.

Tuning into Internal Hunger Cues:

Mindful eating encourages you to listen to your body's internal hunger cues, distinguishing between true hunger and emotional eating. Avoid mindless snacking and eating when not truly hungry.

Slowing Down and Savoring:

Mindful eating emphasizes slowing down and savoring each bite. Put away distractions, focus on the flavors and textures of your food, and appreciate the act of eating.

Honoring Food Choices:

Mindful eating promotes making conscious food choices based on nutrient density, personal preferences, and ethical considerations. Avoid impulsive decisions and prioritize whole, unprocessed foods for optimal nourishment.

Embracing the Sensory Experience:

Mindful eating encourages you to engage all your senses during meals. Notice the visual appeal of your food, the aromas that fill the air, the different textures, and the symphony of flavors dancing on your palate.

Cultivating Gratitude:

Mindful eating fosters an attitude of gratitude for the food that nourishes your body. Reflect on the journey from farm to table and appreciate the hard work of those who contribute to your nourishment.

Overcoming Emotional Eating:

Mindful eating helps you identify and address emotional triggers that lead to overeating. Develop healthy coping mechanisms for stress and emotional challenges to prevent food from becoming an emotional crutch.

Conclusion: Transforming Mealtimes into Moments of Mindfulness

By incorporating mindful eating practices into your Lipocaloric journey, you transform mealtimes into moments of mindfulness, enhancing satiety, deepening your connection with food, and cultivating a healthier relationship with eating. Remember, mindful eating is not about perfection but about cultivating a more conscious and enjoyable approach to nourishing your body and mind.

Part 3

Navigating the Lipocaloric Journey

Chapter 7

Overcoming Challenges and Embracing Sustainable Success

The Lipocaloric Diet, with its profound impact on metabolism and its remarkable health benefits, offers a transformative path to optimal well-being. However, embarking on this journey may present challenges and require a commitment to sustainable practices to achieve long-term success. This chapter delves into the art of overcoming obstacles, maintaining motivation, and cultivating sustainable habits that will support you throughout your Lipocaloric transformation.

Addressing Common Challenges: Navigating the Roadblocks

The Lipocaloric journey, like any significant lifestyle change, may present challenges that can test your resolve and hinder your progress. Recognizing and addressing these challenges proactively is crucial for maintaining motivation and staying on track.

Cravings and Temptations:

Cravings for unhealthy, calorie-dense foods are a common challenge during the initial stages of the Lipocaloric Diet. To combat cravings, focus on nutrient-dense foods that provide sustained satiety. Identify your emotional triggers and develop healthy coping mechanisms to prevent emotional eating.

Plateaus and Weight Loss Stalls:

Weight loss plateaus, where progress seems to stall, can be discouraging. However, it is important to remember that weight loss is not always linear. Continue adhering to the Lipocaloric principles, incorporate more physical activity, and seek guidance from a healthcare professional if needed.

Social Pressures and Dining Out:

Navigating social gatherings and dining out can be challenging while following the Lipocaloric Diet. Make mindful choices when ordering food, focus on nutrient-dense options, and politely decline unhealthy temptations. Practice assertive communication and explain your dietary preferences to others.

Maintaining Motivation and Avoiding Burnout:

Sustaining motivation throughout the Lipocaloric journey is essential for long-term success. Celebrate small victories, focus on non-scale victories such as improved energy levels and better sleep, and seek support from friends, family, or online communities.

Cultivating Sustainable Habits for Lifelong Well-being

Transforming the Lipocaloric Diet into a sustainable lifestyle requires cultivating habits that align with your long-term well-being. These habits will become the foundation for a healthier, happier you.

Incorporating Regular Physical Activity:

Physical activity is an integral part of a sustainable Lipocaloric lifestyle. Find activities you enjoy and gradually increase your activity level. Exercise not only enhances weight loss but also improves overall health and boosts mood.

Prioritizing Sleep:

Adequate sleep is crucial for regulating metabolism, hormones, and overall well-being. Aim for 7-8 hours of quality sleep each night to optimize your body's functioning and support your Lipocaloric journey.

Managing Stress:

Chronic stress can negatively impact metabolism and hinder weight loss efforts. Incorporate stress-management techniques such as yoga, meditation, or spending time in nature into your routine to promote relaxation and overall well-being.

Embracing a Growth Mindset:

Adopting a growth mindset, where you view challenges as opportunities for learning and growth, is essential for sustainable success. Embrace setbacks as temporary learning experiences and maintain a positive outlook on your Lipocaloric journey.

Seeking Professional Guidance:

Don't hesitate to seek guidance from healthcare professionals, registered dietitians, or online communities to gain personalized support and encouragement throughout your Lipocaloric journey.

Conclusion: Embracing a Journey of Transformation

The Lipocaloric Diet, when embraced with a sustainable approach and a growth mindset, offers a transformative path to achieving optimal health and well-being. By overcoming challenges, maintaining motivation, and cultivating healthy habits, you can unlock the remarkable benefits of Lipocalorics and embark on a journey towards a healthier, happier, and more fulfilling life. Remember, sustainability is not about perfection but about progress, adaptability, and a commitment to continuous improvement.

Chapter 8

Unleashing the Power of Exercise: Enhancing the Lipocaloric Experience

Regular physical activity is an integral part of a successful Lipocaloric journey. It enhances weight loss, improves cardiovascular health, boosts energy levels, and promotes muscle maintenance. This chapter delves into the transformative power of exercise, providing guidance on incorporating it seamlessly into your Lipocaloric lifestyle and maximizing its benefits.

Finding Your Exercise Sweet Spot: Discovering Activities You Enjoy

Choosing activities that align with your preferences and fitness level is crucial for maintaining motivation and ensuring long-term adherence to an exercise routine. Explore a variety of options, from brisk walking and cycling to swimming and dancing, to find activities that bring you joy and make exercise a pleasurable experience.

Establishing Realistic Goals and Gradual Progression:

Setting unrealistic exercise goals can lead to discouragement and hinder your progress. Start with achievable goals that align with your current fitness level and gradually increase the intensity and duration of your workouts as you gain strength and endurance.

Incorporating Variety and Avoiding Monotony:

Variety is key to keeping your exercise routine engaging and preventing boredom. Alternate between different activities, incorporate strength training, and explore new fitness classes or outdoor adventures to keep your workouts exciting and challenging.

Maximizing Efficiency with Time-Efficient Exercise:

If time constraints are a concern, consider incorporating high-intensity interval training (HIIT) or circuit training. These time-efficient workouts provide a powerful combination of cardio and strength training, boosting calorie burn and maximizing results in a shorter time frame.

Overcoming Exercise Barriers: Addressing Common Obstacles

Several factors can hinder your motivation to exercise. Recognizing and addressing these barriers proactively can help you maintain consistency and achieve your fitness goals.

Lack of Time:

Schedule your workouts in advance and treat them as important appointments. Prioritize exercise by making it a non-negotiable part of your daily routine, just like brushing your teeth or eating meals.

Lack of Motivation:

Find an exercise buddy or join a fitness class to gain social support and accountability. Set rewards for yourself for achieving exercise milestones, and remind yourself of the long-term benefits of regular physical activity.

Fear of Failure or Judgment:

Remember that everyone starts somewhere. Focus on your own progress, not comparing yourself to others. Celebrate your achievements, no matter how small, and maintain a positive and encouraging mindset.

Exercise and Weight Loss: Understanding the Synergy

While exercise plays a crucial role in weight loss, it is important to understand its synergistic relationship with the Lipocaloric Diet. Exercise enhances calorie expenditure, promotes muscle maintenance, and improves insulin sensitivity, all of which contribute to successful weight loss and improved metabolic health.

Maximizing Weight Loss Benefits:

Pair your Lipocaloric Diet with regular physical activity for optimal weight loss results. Aim for at least 30 minutes of moderate-intensity exercise most days of the week. Gradually increase the intensity and duration of your workouts as your fitness level improves.

Preventing Muscle Loss:

Incorporate strength training exercises at least two to three times per week to maintain muscle mass during weight loss. Muscle burns more calories at rest than fat, contributing to a higher metabolism and enhanced weight loss efforts.

Improving Insulin Sensitivity:

Exercise enhances insulin sensitivity, allowing your body to utilize glucose more efficiently and preventing blood sugar spikes. This improved insulin sensitivity promotes weight loss and reduces the risk of type 2 diabetes.

Conclusion: Unleashing the Transformative Power of Exercise

Incorporating regular physical activity into your Lipocaloric journey is essential for maximizing weight loss, enhancing overall health, and boosting your well-being. By finding activities you enjoy, setting realistic goals, and overcoming common barriers, you can transform exercise into a source of joy and reap the remarkable benefits it has to offer. Remember, consistency is key. Commit to regular workouts, gradually increase your activity level, and embrace the transformative power of exercise as you embark on your Lipocaloric

journey towards a healthier, happier
you.

Chapter 9

Embracing a Holistic Approach to Wellness: Integrating Lifestyle Habits for Optimal Health

The Lipocaloric Diet, while focused on calorie restriction and nutrient density, extends beyond mere dietary choices and encompasses a holistic approach to wellness. This chapter delves into the integration of lifestyle habits that complement the Lipocaloric Diet and promote optimal health and well-being.

Prioritizing Quality Sleep: Restoring and Rejuvenating the Body

Adequate sleep is crucial for optimal physical and mental functioning. Aim for 7-8 hours of quality sleep each night to allow your body to rest, repair, and rejuvenate. Establish a consistent sleep schedule, create a relaxing bedtime routine, and avoid caffeine and electronic devices before bed to promote restful sleep.

Managing Stress Effectively: Fostering Inner Calm and Resilience

Chronic stress can negatively impact metabolism, hindering weight loss efforts and increasing the risk of chronic diseases. Incorporate stress-management techniques such as yoga, meditation, or spending time in nature into your routine to promote relaxation, reduce stress hormones, and enhance overall well-being.

Nurturing Healthy Social Connections: The Power of Human Connection

Social connections play a vital role in overall happiness, well-being, and motivation. Nurture your relationships with friends and family, engage in social activities, and cultivate a supportive network that provides encouragement and accountability throughout your Lipocaloric journey.

Mindful Living: Cultivating Presence and Appreciation

Mindful living involves being present in the moment, savoring experiences, and appreciating the beauty of life. Practice mindfulness techniques such as meditation or deep breathing exercises to reduce stress, enhance self-awareness, and cultivate a sense of inner peace and tranquility.

Seeking Professional Guidance: When to Seek Support

Don't hesitate to seek guidance from healthcare professionals, registered dietitians, or mental health experts if you encounter challenges, experience persistent symptoms, or need personalized support. Their expertise can provide valuable insights, tailored advice, and ongoing support throughout your Lipocaloric journey.

Conclusion: Weaving Lifestyle Habits into the Lipocaloric Tapestry

Integrating healthy lifestyle habits into your Lipocaloric journey is essential for achieving optimal health and well-being. By prioritizing quality sleep, managing stress effectively, nurturing social connections, cultivating mindful living, and seeking professional guidance when needed, you transform the Lipocaloric Diet into a holistic approach to transforming your life. Remember, these lifestyle habits are not mere add-ons but integral components of a comprehensive path to a healthier, happier, and more fulfilling existence

Part 4

Maintaining Success and Beyond

Chapter 10

Maintaining Success: Embracing Long-Term Lifestyle Transformation

The Lipocaloric Diet, with its profound impact on metabolism and its far-reaching health benefits, offers a transformative path to optimal well-being. However, maintaining success and sustaining the positive changes achieved through the Lipocaloric Diet requires a commitment to long-term lifestyle transformation. This chapter delves into strategies for maintaining success, navigating lifestyle adjustments, and cultivating a lifelong love for healthy living.

Understanding the Maintenance Phase: Adapting to a New Normal

The maintenance phase of the Lipocaloric journey involves transitioning from a period of calorie restriction to a sustainable lifestyle that promotes long-term health and well-being. This transition requires gradual adjustments to calorie intake, activity levels, and overall lifestyle habits.

Gradual Calorie Reintroduction:

Reintroduce calories gradually, paying attention to portion sizes, nutrient density, and satiety cues. Avoid drastic increases that could lead to weight regain.

Maintaining Physical Activity:

Continue engaging in regular physical activity, incorporating activities you enjoy and gradually increasing intensity as needed. Exercise is crucial for maintaining weight loss, improving overall health, and boosting energy levels.

Cultivating Healthy Habits:

Integrate the healthy lifestyle habits adopted during the Lipocaloric Diet into your daily routine. Prioritize quality sleep, stress management techniques, mindful living, and strong social connections for long-term well-being.

Addressing Challenges and Relapses:

Expect challenges and setbacks along the way. View them as learning opportunities, not failures. Develop coping mechanisms for emotional eating and seek support from friends, family, or healthcare professionals when needed.

Embracing a Lifelong Love for Healthy Living:

Shift your mindset from a temporary diet to a lifelong commitment to healthy living. View healthy choices as an investment in your well-being, not as restrictions. Find joy in nourishing your body and mind, and appreciate the transformative power of a healthy lifestyle.

Conclusion: Embarking on a Journey of Perpetual Transformation

Maintaining success with the Lipocaloric Diet is not about reaching a destination but about embarking on a journey of perpetual transformation. It is about cultivating a lifelong love for healthy living, embracing a holistic approach to well-being, and continuously adapting to the changing needs of your body and mind. Remember, sustainable success lies in finding balance, flexibility, and a deep-rooted appreciation for the transformative power of healthy living

Chapter 11

Celebrating Success and Sharing Your Journey

Achieving success with the Lipocaloric Diet and transforming your lifestyle is a remarkable accomplishment worthy of celebration. This chapter delves into the importance of recognizing your achievements, sharing your journey with others, and inspiring others to embrace a healthier path.

Acknowledging Your Achievements: Honoring Your Hard Work

Take time to acknowledge your progress, no matter how small. Celebrate reaching milestones, achieving weight loss goals, and adopting healthier habits. Recognizing your achievements reinforces positive behavior and fuels motivation to continue on your journey.

Sharing Your Journey: Inspiring Others Through Your Story

Sharing your Lipocaloric experience with others can have a profound impact, providing inspiration, support, and practical insights for those considering embarking on a similar journey. Share your story through personal accounts, online forums, or support groups, offering valuable guidance and encouragement.

Empowering Others: Becoming a Beacon of Healthy Living

As you progress on your Lipocaloric journey, you may find yourself becoming a beacon of healthy living, inspiring others to adopt healthier habits and make positive changes in their own lives. Share your knowledge, offer support, and encourage others to embrace a holistic approach to well-being.

Becoming a Healthy Living Advocate:

Your Lipocaloric journey can extend beyond personal transformation and inspire broader change. Consider becoming a healthy living advocate, promoting awareness about the Lipocaloric Diet, educating others about nutrition and lifestyle habits, and supporting initiatives that promote public health and well-being.

Conclusion: A Legacy of Inspiration and Well-being

Your success with the Lipocaloric Diet is not just about you; it is a testament to your resilience, determination, and commitment to a healthier life. As you celebrate your achievements and share your journey with others, you leave a legacy of inspiration, empowering others to embrace a healthier path and transforming the lives of those around you. Remember, your story has the power to inspire, guide, and motivate others to embark on their own journeys towards optimal health and well-being.

Chapter 12

Embracing the Lipocaloric Lifestyle: A Tapestry of Transformation

The Lipocaloric Diet, with its profound impact on cellular metabolism and its far-reaching health benefits, offers a transformative path to optimal health and well-being. This chapter culminates the journey, reflecting on the holistic approach to transformation, the significance of personal growth, and the enduring impact of adopting a healthy lifestyle.

A Tapestry of Transformation: Weaving Together the Threads of Change

The Lipocaloric Diet is not merely a dietary approach; it is a tapestry of transformation, weaving together the threads of nutrition, lifestyle habits, and mindset shifts. It is a journey that encompasses not just physical changes but also mental and emotional growth.

Nourishing the Body and Mind: A Holistic Approach to Well-being

The Lipocaloric Diet extends beyond mere calorie restriction and nutrient density. It encourages a holistic approach to well-being, encompassing regular physical activity, adequate sleep, effective stress management, and mindful living practices. These interconnected elements contribute to optimal physical health, mental clarity, and emotional resilience.

Cultivating Personal Growth: Embracing Challenges as Opportunities

The Lipocaloric journey is not without its challenges. However, these challenges provide opportunities for personal growth, fostering resilience, adaptability, and a deeper understanding of oneself. Overcoming obstacles strengthens the resolve to stay on track, enhancing self-belief and fueling motivation.

A Ripple Effect of Change: Inspiring Others to Embrace a Healthier Path

As you transform your own life through the Lipocaloric Diet, you have the potential to inspire others to embrace a healthier path. Your story, shared with honesty and compassion, can motivate others to make positive changes in their own lives, creating a ripple effect of well-being that extends beyond your immediate circle.

The Enduring Legacy of a Healthier Lifestyle: A Gift to Yourself and Others

The Lipocaloric Diet, once embraced, becomes a lifelong gift to yourself and others. It is a commitment to optimal health, a dedication to self-care, and a testament to the power of continuous improvement. As you continue to nourish your body and mind, you empower others to do the same, creating a legacy of well-being that enriches your life and the lives of those around you.

Conclusion: A Journey of Transformation and Inspiration

The Lipocaloric Diet is a journey of transformation, a pathway to optimal health, and a source of inspiration for others. It is a testament to the human capacity for change, the power of resilience, and the enduring impact of a healthy lifestyle. As you continue on this journey, remember that every step forward, every challenge overcome, and every moment of self-discovery contributes to a life of vitality, well-being, and profound fulfillment.

Part 5

Reflections and Insights

Chapter 13

Embracing the Lipocaloric Lifestyle: A Journey of Self-Discovery and Lifelong Wellness

The Lipocaloric Diet, with its emphasis on calorie restriction, nutrient density, and a holistic approach to well-being, offers a transformative path to optimal health and a deeper understanding of oneself. This concluding chapter delves into the profound impact of the Lipocaloric journey, highlighting the significance of self-discovery, the importance of lifelong wellness, and the transformative power of embracing a healthy lifestyle.

A Journey of Self-Discovery: Unveiling Your Inner Strength and Potential

The Lipocaloric journey is not merely about achieving physical transformation; it is a profound exploration of one's inner strength, resilience, and potential. As you navigate challenges, overcome obstacles, and make conscious choices that align with your well-being, you uncover a deeper understanding of yourself, your values, and your capacity for change.

Embracing Lifelong Wellness: A Commitment to Continuous Improvement

The Lipocaloric Diet serves as a catalyst for lifelong wellness, instilling habits and practices that extend far beyond weight loss. By prioritizing nutrient-dense foods, incorporating regular physical activity, and embracing stress-management techniques, you cultivate a holistic approach to well-being that supports you throughout your life.

Transforming Your Relationship with Food: Cultivating Mindful Eating and Appreciation

The Lipocaloric journey transforms your relationship with food, shifting from mere sustenance to a mindful and appreciative experience. You learn to savor the flavors, textures, and nutritional value of food, fostering a healthier mindset and a deeper connection with the nourishment you provide your body.

Inspiring Others to Embrace a Healthier Path: Sharing Your Story and Empowering Others

As you progress on your Lipocaloric journey, you become a beacon of inspiration, encouraging others to adopt healthier habits and make positive changes in their own lives. Sharing your story, offering support, and advocating for well-being have the power to ripple outwards, creating a community of individuals committed to a healthier lifestyle.

A Legacy of Well-being: A Gift to Yourself and the World

The Lipocaloric journey leaves a lasting legacy of well-being, not just for you but for those around you. Your transformation serves as a testament to the power of self-belief, the importance of prioritizing health, and the transformative impact of a healthy lifestyle.

Conclusion: Embracing the Journey and Celebrating the Transformative Power of Wellness

The Lipocaloric Diet is an empowering journey of self-discovery, a path to lifelong wellness, and a source of inspiration for others. It is a testament to the human capacity for change, the power of resilience, and the enduring impact of embracing a healthy lifestyle. As you continue on this transformational path, remember that every step forward, every challenge overcome, and every moment of self-discovery contributes to a life of vitality, well-being, and profound fulfillment. Embrace the journey, celebrate the transformative power of wellness, and continue to inspire others to unlock their own potential for optimal health and a life brimming with vitality and joy.

Conclusion

A Tapestry of Transformation and Inspiration

The Lipocaloric Diet, with its profound impact on cellular metabolism and its far-reaching health benefits, offers a transformative path to optimal health and a deeper understanding of oneself. Throughout this book, we have explored the intricacies of the Lipocaloric Diet, delved into its scientific underpinnings, and witnessed its transformative impact on the lives of individuals like Sarah.

As we conclude this journey, we carry with us a profound understanding that the Lipocaloric Diet is not merely a dietary approach; it is a tapestry of transformation, woven together with threads of nutrition, lifestyle habits, and mindset shifts. It is a journey that encompasses not just physical changes but also mental and emotional growth.

The Lipocaloric Diet extends beyond calorie restriction and nutrient density. It encourages a holistic approach to well-being, encompassing regular physical activity, adequate sleep, effective stress management, and mindful living practices. These interconnected elements contribute to optimal physical health, mental clarity, and emotional resilience.

The Lipocaloric journey is not without its challenges. However, these challenges provide opportunities for personal growth, fostering resilience, adaptability, and a deeper understanding of oneself. Overcoming obstacles strengthens the resolve to stay on track, enhancing self-belief and fueling motivation.

As you transform your life through the Lipocaloric Diet, you have the potential to inspire others to embrace a healthier path. Your story, shared with honesty and compassion, can motivate others to make positive changes in their own lives, creating a ripple effect of well-being that extends beyond your immediate circle.

The Lipocaloric Diet is a journey of self-discovery, a path to lifelong wellness, and a source of inspiration for others. It is a testament to the human capacity for change, the power of resilience, and the enduring impact of a healthy lifestyle. As you continue on this transformational path, remember that every step forward, every challenge overcome, and every moment of self-discovery contributes to a life of vitality, well-being, and profound fulfillment.

Embrace the journey, celebrate the transformative power of wellness, and continue to inspire others to unlock their own potential for optimal health and a life brimming with vitality and joy.